Wellness Shots R

CW01082980

Learn Powerful F
Wellness Shots to E
Health and Wellbeing

Temmy Miller

Table of Contents

Introduction

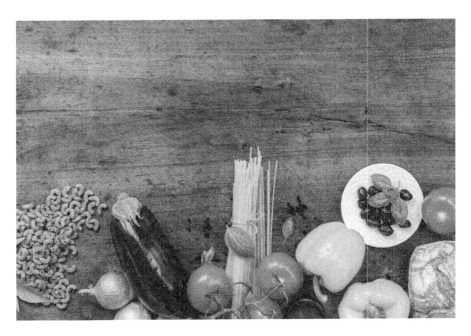

Our health as we know it is highly significant, it is a great factor in our lives and is a gift handed to us to take care of. We may not know it, or we may not care, but being healthy is one of the greatest contributions that you can give to your life.

Being healthy is one phenomenon that is followed all around the world, and if some people do not follow it, then they should immediately start adhering to it. Keeping our minds and bodies healthy is one way of knowing that whatever we do in life and wherever we go we will be okay.

Our well-being counts on the way we treat ourselves, not only that, but it counts on all the factors that contribute to keeping our body and mind the way they are. When we think about our health, we look at our diet, our activities, and the thoughts that run through our heads.

Our opinions may dishearten us to do things and also may create certain illnesses that last a long time. Abusing food can lead us to be obese and also makes us lazy, and all the wrong activities may prevent us from being healthy and may stop us from experiencing different things.

Our emotions play a huge role in us feeling well, they are the stimulants that help us feel a certain way. Not only that, but they can also determine how we view life and how we think about different things. Our well-being is like our happiness, it is a factor that is equal to being positive.

We may talk about all the positive things that we do in our life, which boost our energy and keep us energized and we may also talk about all the other things that take care of our health both mentally and physically.

However, the element that is emphasized is wellness doses, which are more of which improve our physical well-being in our lives and are something that not many people follow. People either don't want to or don't like to do these things, or they are too busy to do so.

Many people claim to have skincare routines and heavy exercises that help keep their bodies looking healthy and fit, but these factors only last for a certain amount of time. What matters more than the inner workings of our bodies?

If we apply this technique of having such recipes in our daily lives, we will gain numerous benefits. These may range from staying healthy to also being efficient in the work we do, there is an obvious need for people to stay healthy in today's world. A person's weight doesn't matter, what matters is that our body is healthy.

To keep our bodies healthy, we, on our own, should take the necessary initiatives and keep ourselves fit and healthy.

Implementing these wellness shots in our life is something everyone should do. The taste shouldn't matter in front of the benefits and to achieve benefits, everyone needs to work a little harder.

There are some things we attempt in life for our benefit, and there are times when all we want to do is stay healthy. This can be achieved by having these wellness shots consumed in our life. There are many failures in our lives and there are many times when achieving things gets a bit hard. Keeping ourselves happy and taking care of our bodies and minds is one such aspect that might assist us in completing any further difficult work.

Not only that, but wellness shots have seemed to play a vital role in many people's lives and they may continue doing so if they are given the time to intake and also appreciated, not only by the person themselves but also by the body on the effect that they have on it.

Chapter 1: Detox Wellness Shots Recipes

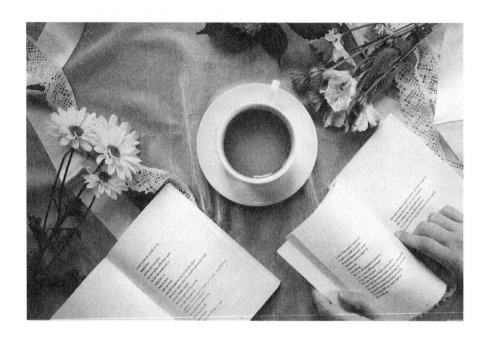

Apple Cider Vinegar Tonic

Because numerous helpful components are employed in the process of manufacturing this shot, which provides the proper quantity of nourishment for health benefits, this type of tonic is mostly designed for weight reduction.

Apple cider vinegar has a sour taste which may help a person eat less but stay content with what they consume, instead of thinking about what they cannot. It even has zero calories, making it a popular weight-loss substance.

Green tea, which is also used in the recipe, has the components of caffeine and antioxidants which boost fat loss. Ginger is one other ingredient that burns calories, and maple syrup is known to sweeten the drink, making it natural and consumable.

It is believed to be the most popular among those who wish to lose weight, and it can be adopted by taking a shot of it frequently or even on occasion, but it is known to be more effective when used consistently.

- **Time:** 5 minutes
- **Serving Size:** 1 cup
- **Nutritional Facts:**
  - Calories 22
  - Carbohydrates 5 g
  - Sugars 4.1 g
  - Vitamin C 0.1 mg
  - Folate 0.2 mg
  - Calcium 8.2 mg
  - Iron 0.1 mg
  - Magnesium 3 mg
  - Potassium 58.3 mg
  - Sodium 1.8 mg
  - Added Sugar 4 g

Ingredients:

- 1 cup brewed chilled green tea
- 1 tbsp raw cider vinegar
- 1 tsp pure maple syrup
- 1 tsp grated fresh ginger
- 1 lemon wedge

Directions:

1. Stir the green tea (chilled), vinegar, syrup, and ginger in a medium glass thoroughly.
2. Add a squeeze of lemon if desired.

Hot Lemon Ginger Detox Tonic

This recipe is required to be implemented in our daily morning routines as it improves hydration and makes the body naturally detox. Ginger is also known to be great for digestion, it can protect our body from various diseases while also contributing to skin health. It helps keep our skin healthy and shiny.

Both lemon and ginger have high immunity-boosting properties, while ginger is also known to reduce the risks of some cancers. A sufficient amount taken every day is enough to keep the body healthy and boost immunity along with all the other nutrition we acquire from food daily.

It's a beneficiary routine that can be followed by many since it even helps with both treating and preventing the flu.

As a recipe shortcut, honey, lemon, and a knob of ginger can be added to the blender with hot water and taken out when frothy.

It is also recommended to make a big batch of it and store it in the fridge and take amounts while heating it on the stove, then repeat the process when it is finished.

Raw honey is a preferred ingredient, but it can also be added according to our level of desired sweetness.

- **Time:** 15 minutes
- **Serving Size:** 2 cups
- **Prep Time:** 5 minutes

- **Cook Time:** 10 minutes
- **Nutritional Facts:**
  - Calories 71
  - Sugar 18 g
  - Sodium 0 mg
  - Fat 0 g
  - Saturated Fat 0 g
  - Unsaturated Fat 0 g
  - Trans Fat 0 g
  - Carbohydrates 19 g
  - Fiber 0 g
  - Protein 0 g
  - Cholesterol 0 mg

Ingredients:

- 1½ cup water
- 2 pieces of fresh peeled ginger
- ½ juiced lemon
- 2 tbsp raw honey

Directions:

1. On the side with the largest holes, grate the ginger on the box grater.
2. In a small saucepan, add the grated ginger, lemon juice, and honey.
3. Bring it to a simmer for about five minutes.

4. Pour the lemon ginger tonic into a blender and blend on low until frothy.

5. Pour into a mug of the desired size and enjoy the benefits.

Ginger Lemon and Cayenne Shot

Ginger is typically known for its ability to transform a savory dish due to its unique and spicy flavor. It is also known to have some of the best nutrients and compounds that are beneficial for both our mind and body's well-being.

Paired with the powerful antioxidant properties of cayenne, both these ingredients in one shot are guaranteed to provide a boost of energy whenever and wherever we need it. Even if we do have a healthy balanced diet filled with all sorts of nutrients and properties that claim to be useful and needed in our lives, having a boost in the form of a shot that has all the required nutrients and more is beneficial and may aid us in replenishing our energy.

Research even suggests that consuming powerful ingredients like ginger in the form of liquid helps us reap all of the nutritional benefits that ginger has to offer.

Ginger, which is also an anti-inflammatory, is utilized in a variety of medicinal practices to lower inflammation and can be used to treat illness and improve cognitive function. The ginger root is preferred over the dry powder form because it has more nutrients and the oils added to it are helpful to our health.

It is an additional supplement that many people prefer to consume and is allegedly also advised in health care procedures for lowering blood pressure. Cayenne is often found to reduce hunger levels and boost metabolism. When used in a meal, it is also believed to increase the body temperatures which results in its consumption burning calories.

It aids in various ailments as well, cayenne has been known to have its high nutritional value and benefits, but, when combined with ginger, it is known to be an effective mixture.

Lemon is known to be an excellent source of vitamin C. Due to its high vitamin quantity, the lemon in this recipe acts as a powerful antioxidant that helps balance the spicy ginger flavor while also cleaning the digestive system and maintaining the body's pH level. It even provides integrity to the skin helping it stay healthy, while its powerful antioxidants and refreshing taste add uniqueness to the mixture.

Turmeric is also known to be from the same root family as cayenne. It has various health benefits and is also used in many medicinal practices. Even if turmeric comes in many different forms, including powder, it is advised the turmeric used for this recipe be fresh, raw turmeric which can aid a person in reaping the complete benefits present in it.

- **Time:** 10 minutes
- **Serving Size:** 4 cups
- **Prep Time:** 5 minutes
- **Cook Time:** 5 minutes
- **Nutritional Facts:**
    - Calories 15
    - Sugar 3 g
    - Sodium 0 mg
    - Fat 0 g
    - Carbohydrates 4 g

- o   Fiber 0 g
- o   Protein 0 g

Ingredients:

- 2 sliced lemons
- ½ inch fresh ginger piece
- ½ inch raw turmeric root or ¼ tsp of turmeric powder
- ¼ tsp of cayenne powder

Directions:

1. Combine the lemon and the piece of ginger through a juicer.
2. If raw turmeric root is used, this will be combined with the other ingredients too.
3. Strain the juice through a sieve or mesh strainer.
4. The lemon juice can be extracted by hand too, and the ginger can also be squeezed to let the juice out as much as possible through the mesh strainer or whatever equipment is being used to do so.
5. Stir the lemon juice into the ginger juice.
6. Stir the cayenne powder in the drink at last. If turmeric root is not being used, add turmeric powder with the cayenne powder and stir the drink making it ready to consume.
7. Take the shot, and feel its kick!

Wheatgrass Shot

Wheatgrass shots are packed with high levels of vitamins and minerals. It also contains the eight kinds of amino acids that our bodies can't produce on their own. The juice or the shot can also help with improving respiratory function.

Other functions like aiding in weight loss, preventing inflammation, controlling blood sugar levels, and easing a sore throat are also benefits of consuming wheatgrass shots. When wheatgrass juice is first consumed, it may cause side effects like stomachache, headache, fatigue, and nausea.

It is a powerful detox and, hence, needs time adjusting. Adjusting this can be easier by starting with smaller amounts of juice, even adding it to other recipes to keep it diluted is beneficiary.

It is recommended to drink a wheatgrass shot in the early mornings, especially on an empty stomach, and wait an hour or two before eating anything else, this method can also help with nausea. The juice can also be put to use for the skin, to soothe scars or bite marks, and more.

- **Time:** 10 minutes
- **Serving Size:** 1 cup
- **Prep Time:** 5 minutes
- **Cook Time:** 5 minutes
- **Nutritional Facts:**
  - Calories 188
  - Carbohydrates 45 g
  - Protein 8 g
  - Fiber 30 g

- Protein 1 g
- Fat 0 g
- Sodium 0 g
- Vitamin K 86 mcg

Ingredients:

10½ oz fresh wheatgrass

Directions:

1. Cut the wheatgrass as low as possible to the root before juicing it, or it should be ensured that it is cut precisely if bought.
2. Rinse the wheatgrass and discard any leaves that seemed to have turned yellow.
3. Pass small bunches of it through the juicer, and the pulp residue may form continuously. Removing it manually is the best solution.
4. When done, the juice will be all that is remaining with the small amount of leftover pulp.

Chapter 2: Turmeric Wellness Shots Recipes

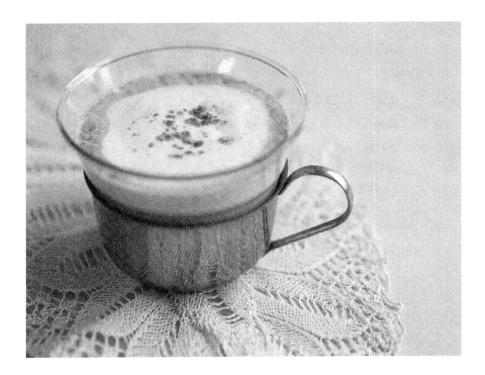

Simple Turmeric Shot

Turmeric is known to be a miracle spice, all due to a compound named curcumin present in it. It acts as a powerful antioxidant while at the same time helping with lowering the level of enzymes that cause inflammation, which is the root of most diseases.

The antioxidants present help in fighting off free radicals in the body and can act as a boost when our body can't produce them on its own. It also helps in boosting brain function which helps grow the brain and keeps it from age-related brain diseases.

The main active ingredient of turmeric even acts as an anti-depressant which helps boost happy hormones and can also help delay aging. It benefits the skin in various ways, it heals wounds, brightens the dark circles, and even keeps the skin glowing which makes it look healthier and makes a person feel much younger.

The use of powdered turmeric can also be done instead of the turmeric roots. These turmeric shots can be made in batches and stored in the refrigerator. Even so, they need to be finished before four days are up since the wellness power in them begins to fade with time.

- **Time:** 10 minutes
- **Serving Size:** 1 cup
- **Prep Time:** 5 minutes
- **Cook Time:** 5 minutes
- **Nutritional Facts:**
  - Calories 119
  - Carbohydrates 22 g
  - Protein 3 g
  - Fat 3 g
  - Saturated Fat 1 g
  - Sodium 12 mg
  - Potassium 810 mg
  - Fiber 6 g
  - Sugar 3 g
  - Vitamin A 61 mg
  - Vitamin C 23 mg
  - Calcium 59 mg

o   Iron 12 mg

Ingredients:

- ½ cup squeezed orange juice
- ¼ cup coconut water
- 4 roots of fresh chopped turmeric
- ¼ tsp black pepper

Directions:

1. Chop the turmeric and juice the oranges.
2. Add the chopped turmeric, the black pepper, and the juice of the oranges to a high or medium-speed blender until the mixture is smooth and no clumps are visible.
3. Strain the mixture to get rid of any additional paper skin of the root or the orange pulp.
4. Drink your shot.

Ginger Turmeric Shot

Ginger and turmeric are two such ingredients that are highly effective and highly favored by many. Their immunity-solving capabilities and pain-relieving properties are known to be quite favorable, especially the people who may face a lot of pain during sickness or menstrual cycles.

Both these ingredients contribute to better skin health and are barriers to various chronic diseases. They can also be taken as an alternative to caffeine, especially in the mornings when the bold flavor of the shot kicks in along with other boosting variables.

Even known to be a great source of vitamin C, which helps with the metabolism of the body, nothing better to take on a busy day. They can support our health and are fairly easy to add to our diets. One plus or bonus factor is their good flavor, which makes drinking it easy and sufficient.

These shots can be prepared and stored in the refrigerator for about two weeks, before consumption.

- **Time:** 15 minutes
- **Serving Size:** 4 cups
- **Prep Time:** 5 minutes
- **Cook Time:** 10 minutes

Ingredients:

- 1 knob of fresh grated and peeled turmeric or 2 tsp ground turmeric powder
- 1 knob of peeled and grated ginger
- 3 ground cardamom pods
- 4 cups water
- ¼ cup freshly squeezed lemon juice
- 2 tbsp honey
- ¼ tsp of freshly ground pepper to taste

Directions:

1. Combine the grated turmeric, ginger, ground cardamom, black pepper, and two cups of water in a saucepan over medium-low heat.
2. Simmer for 8-10 minutes until fragrant.
3. Strain through a fine mesh strainer into a lidded heat-proof container.
4. In a separate container, whisk honey and lemon juice together.
5. Add the mixture to the turmeric mixture along with the leftover two cups of water.
6. Refrigerate until chilled.

Beetroot Turmeric Shot

A beetroot shot enables a person to consume a lot of essential vitamins and nutrients in one go. It offers a wide range of health benefits and can also be implemented into our lives easier through a routine.

As turmeric has proven to be nature's most potent ingredient, its mixture with beetroot makes the shot highly nutritious, an amazing source of magnesium, and can also help support the healthy functions of the body, which may include the promotion of easy blood flow and our digestive health.

These also protect the body from inflammation, hence keeping it away from various diseases which could affect the body negatively. These shots if taken into a routine will automatically be a known necessity in our life, especially when the effects take place and the person starts feeling healthier.

If the taste is still not good enough, you can try adding apple slices or a spoonful of honey to enhance it.

- **Time:** 15 minutes
- **Serving Size:** 2 cups
- **Prep Time:** 10 minutes
- **Cook Time:** 5 minutes

Ingredients:

- 4 cups of cubed and deseeded watermelons
- 2 medium beets
- ¼ cup grated ginger root
- ¼ grated turmeric root
- 1 medium lemon
- 1 cup of ice cubes

Directions:

1. Chop the beetroot into small, thin slices for it to go through the juicer/blender.
2. Remove the outer rind of the lemon, and chop the flesh into slices ensuring there are no pips.
3. Put one half to the side, while gradually adding the other half into the blender.
4. Along with the lemon, add the watermelon and beetroot, blending until smooth.
5. Then, add the grated ginger and turmeric, along with the ice cubes.
6. When the mixture is done, ensure that there are no lumps left behind.

7. Taste the juice and determine if it needs more lemon. If it does, add the remaining lemon that was kept to the side.

8. If not, store it in the fridge where it will stay fresh for three to four days.

Ginger Turmeric Carrot Shot

There are many benefits when consuming carrots. They are a full storehouse of nutrients that have their own properties and qualities. And, in many other cases, the carrot is a vegetable that is enjoyed by many.

Among its many properties, the one that it is mainly known for is improving eyesight. They are rich in substances like lutein and lycopene which help in maintaining good eyesight and even night vision.

Carrots aid in weight loss. Since they contain fibers, it is easily known to help with achieving weight loss since the fibers cause fullness which prevents a person from eating any other food that could inhibit weight loss.

It helps in ensuring the body's proper digestion. It helps with boosting heart health. It helps in lowering blood pressure, since potassium, which is present in carrots, helps the smooth flow of blood and brings down high blood pressure levels. It helps with boosting our skin, making it glow, and it helps in boosting our immunity as a whole.

Ginger and turmeric are two spices to be consumed regularly. They could even be taken with different combinations of food since they help in enhancing taste with their unique flavors. They also are known to have many properties like turmeric, which is known to improve brain function and reduce inflammation. Similarly, ginger has properties that help with digestion and relieve nausea.

- **Time:** 15 minutes
- **Serving Size:** 4 shots
- **Prep Time:** 5 minutes
- **Cook Time:** 10 minutes
- **Nutritional Facts:**
    - 59 Calories, Protein 1.3 g
    - Carbohydrates 13.7 g
    - Dietary Fiber 3.3 g
    - Sugars 7.2 g, Fat 0.4 g
    - Saturated Fat 0.1 g
    - Vitamin A 12618 IU
    - Vitamin C 11.4 mg
    - Folate 21.9 mg
    - Calcium 42.2 mg
    - Iron 0.5 mg
    - Magnesium 17.9 mg
    - Potassium 470.6 mg
    - Sodium 127.1 mg

Ingredients:

- 1 pound of coarsely chopped carrots
- 1 piece of fresh peeled turmeric chopped into pieces
- 1 piece of fresh peeled ginger chopped into pieces
- ¾ cup unsweetened coconut water

- A pinch of salt

Directions:

1. Combine the carrots, turmeric, and ginger along with half a cup of unsweetened cup of coconut water and blend it at a high speed.
2. When smooth enough, pour the mixture through a fine mesh strainer into a storage vessel, a jug, or a bowl… whichever is preferred.
3. Get rid of the solid remains.
4. Stir in the salt and the remaining ¼ cup of coconut water and drink when ready!

Chapter 3: Fruit Wellness Shots Recipes

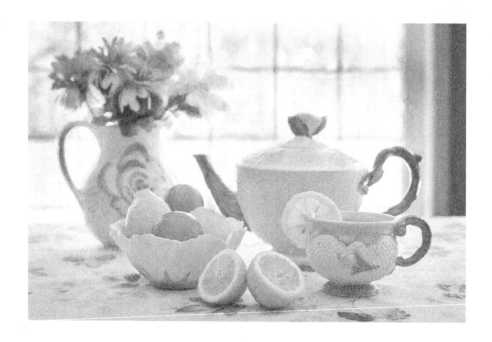

Banana & Spinach Elixir Shot

Green elixir is known to be an all-in-one supplement that helps nourish the body wholly with the world's most powerful nutrients added into the making of it. Due to all the natural ingredients added to it, it is essentially packed with vitamins, minerals, and antioxidants, which protect our bodies from accumulating oxidative stress and enable them to function well.

It boosts energy and mood, fights premature aging and balances, and increases the right amount of alkalinity. Coconut oil is filled with medium chain-filled fatty acids which our body can easily use for energy, as well as maca which is a natural energy booster.

Iron in spinach is a key factor in avoiding fatigue. These ingredients and their nutrients should be consumed before a busy day, to keep your energy up for hours.

Using half coconut milk and half almond milk is recommended. For a thicker juice, frozen banana slices are added.

- **Time:** 10 minutes
- **Serving Size:** 6 small cups or 1 cup
- **Prep Time:** 5 minutes
- **Cook Time:** 5 minutes
- **Nutritional Facts:**
  - Calories 191
  - Sugar 5.3 g
  - Fat 14.9 g
  - Carbohydrates 11.1 g
  - Fiber 1.5 g
  - Protein 2.9 g

Ingredients:

- 1 ripe banana, cut into slices
- 1 tbsp almond butter
- 2 cups fresh spinach
- 2-3 mint leaves to taste
- 2 tsp freshly grated ginger
- ½ inch fresh turmeric (skin removed)
- 3 tbsp yogurt
- 1 tbsp ground flax seeds

- 1 tsp maca powder
- 1 tbsp coconut oil
- ¾ cup coconut milk

Directions:

1. Add all the ingredients with their specified amounts to a blender.
2. Blend on high speed until smooth for 1 minute.
3. Divide and serve into regular or shot glasses.
4. Serve immediately or refrigerate for a few hours before consumption.

Cherry & Pomegranate Shot

Tart cherry juice improves workout performance and also helps in sleeping better. Our strength gain may increase and this shot may provide relief after intense exercise, especially when our muscles are sore and aching. Some researchers have found that regularly consuming tart cherry juice may improve one's cognitive abilities.

These shots may also promote brain health The antioxidants and other positive compounds may have protective effects on the brain cells and these also strengthen our immune system considerably if taken regularly.

Tart cherry juice is filled with more nutrients than its powder. It should be drunk with caution since the sugar molecule active in the drink can cause stomachache or diarrhea for some. Overall, its benefits are many, and if regularly implemented it is a great supplement booster.

- **Time:** 10 minutes
- **Serving Size:** 8 shot glasses
- **Prep Time:** 5 minutes
- **Cook Time:** 5 minutes
- **Nutritional Facts:**
  - Calories 43
  - Protein 0.6 g
  - Carbohydrates 10.3g
  - Dietary Fiber 0.1 g
  - Sugars 9.6 g
  - Fat 0.1 g
  - Vitamin A 100.9IU
  - Vitamin C 2.3 mg
  - Folate 6.1 mg
  - Calcium 15.3 mg
  - Iron 0.3 mg
  - Magnesium 2.7 mg
  - Potassium 146.6 mg
  - Sodium 17.8 mg

Ingredients:

- 2 cups tart cherry juice
- ½ cup pomegranate arils
- ⅓ cup fresh basil leaves
- 2 tbsp orange juice

Directions:

1. Combine the cherry juice, pomegranate arils, basil, and orange juice in the blender.
2. Blend it on high speed until smooth.
3. Place a strainer over a glass jar, and let it seep through a cheesecloth and into the storage container.
4. Once all the liquid is strained, discard the solids.
5. Cover and refrigerate the shots until chilled for about 15 minutes and drink.

Apple, Spinach & Lemon Shot

Spinach is a vegetable that is beneficial for skin, hair, and bone health. It also provides different nutrients, including vitamins and minerals, which are beneficial to the body. The other possible health benefits that spinach has include improving blood glucose levels which helps with control for people with diabetes, lowering the risk of cancer, and increasing bone health when consumed.

Spinach is not only nutritious but also a plant-based source of iron. Spinach contains calcium which we consume when we drink the recipe, but this sort of calcium would be harder to absorb by the body than the dairy-sourced calcium.

It also contains magnesium which is necessary for energy metabolism, maintaining muscle and nerve function, keeping your heartbeats regulated, achieving a healthy immune system, and maintaining blood pressure.

It also helps with asthma management, lowering blood pressure, and promoting digestive regularity. It helps us provide vitamin A which moderates the oil production in the skin pores and in our hair follicles, which helps in moisturizing both the skin and hair, keeping them shiny and healthy.

Apples, too, are a good source of different healthy nutrients and vitamins. The main components of having an apple may include feeling full and reducing the body's calorie intake. It may also help boost blood sugar control, heart health, cancer prevention, and brain function.

Apple should be especially involved in our balanced diet as it has loads of benefits and is hard to dislike the taste of. Its aid in weight loss is also one reason why people may decide to consume it. Taking this shot daily and regularly is important and can benefit our health in ways that we may not expect.

- **Time:** 10 minutes
- **Serving Size:** 4 shots
- **Prep Time:** 5 minutes
- **Cook Time:** 5 minutes
- **Nutritional Facts:**
  - Calories 45
  - Protein 0.9 g
  - Carbohydrates 11 g
  - Sugars 7.8 g
  - Fat 0.2 g
  - Vitamin A 1545.2 IU
  - Vitamin C 17.6 mg
  - Folate 41.8 mg
  - Calcium 32.7 mg
  - Iron 0.5 mg

- o   Magnesium 21.3 mg
- o   Potassium 310.9 mg
- o   Sodium 48.5 mg

Ingredients:

- 1 sliced medium apple
- 2 cups fresh spinach
- 3 roughly chopped stalks of celery
- 1 cup coconut water
- 3 tbsp lemon juice

Directions:

1. Combine the sliced apple, spinach, celery, coconut water, and lemon juice into a blender.
2. Blend them on high speed until smooth.
3. Arrange a layer of cheesecloth on a shallow bowl or large glass jar.
4. Pour the mixture into the strainer to let the liquid seep into the storage vessel.
5. Once all the liquid is strained, discard the solids that remain.
6. Cover and refrigerate the shots until chilled for up to 15 minutes or even one week, whichever is preferable.

Elderberry & Cinnamon Shot

The berries and the flowers of elderberry are packed with various nutrients, vitamins, and antioxidants that may help in boosting our immune systems, helping in taming inflammation, lessening stress, and protecting our hearts.

The elderberries are also used by many experts for preventing and easing cold and flu symptoms. Since it also is considered to be the world's most healing plant, it has many other treatments which help benefit a person:

- They help in aiding and preventing constipation
- They aid against certain infections that could interrupt or affect our breathing
- They can help prevent headaches and fever, as they help heal and keep our bodies safe from them
- They can prevent various kidney problems
- They help in easing minor skin conditions and are especially resistant to stress

Even though it is known to be a medicinal plant, many side effects come from it. This is especially true when eating raw berries, which can cause vomiting, diarrhea, or nausea. A pregnant woman shouldn't be taking it.

Unlike the berries and the flowers, the other parts of the plant such as the twigs, seeds, and leaves are known to be toxic and should be avoided at all costs. People with immunity problems may have a reaction to it, and, if a person accumulates a rash or breathing problem after eating it, they may be allergic to it.

It's better to consult a doctor or medical professional before taking elderberries since there are advantages as well as disadvantages that can affect a person's health in different ways.

The mixture in this recipe should be warm, not burning hot. It is recommended to take one tablespoon of it daily, but if taking it with a spoon is not sufficient enough, it can be added to a smoothie mix or even taken with sparkling water. This specific mixture must especially be taken when a person gets the flu or gets symptoms of it.

- **Time:** 35 minutes
- **Serving Size:** 3 cups
- **Prep Time:** 5 minutes
- **Cook Time:** 30 minutes
- **Nutritional Facts:**
  - Calories 375
  - Carbohydrates 101 g
  - Sodium 20 mg
  - Potassium 160 mg
  - Fiber 3 g
  - Sugar 92 g
  - Vitamin A 220IU
  - Vitamin C 13.6 mg
  - Calcium 40 mg
  - Iron 1.3 mg

Ingredients:

- 4 cups dried elderberries
- 3 cups of water
- 1 cinnamon stick
- 1 tsp ground ginger

- 4 whole cloves
- 1 cup honey

Directions:

1. Combine the berries, water, cloves, ginger, and cinnamon stick in a large pot.
2. Put to boil.
3. Once set on boiling, allow the berry mixture to simmer. Let it simmer for 30 minutes.
4. After the 30 minutes are up, remove the pot from the heat.
5. Strain the mixture through a cheesecloth or sieve over a bowl or jar, whichever is more preferred.
6. Push the berries into the strainer with a wooden spoon to squeeze out the extra juice.
7. When done, get rid of the solid remains while stirring honey into the mixture, and enjoy while only slightly warm.

Chapter 4: Being Well VS Being Unwell

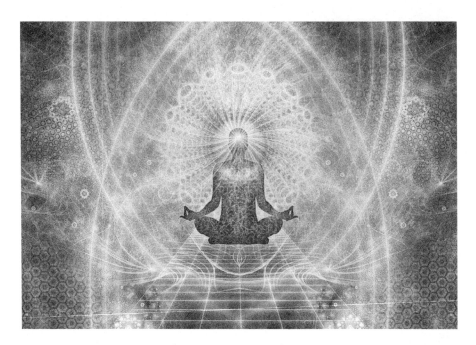

It is a form of temporary illness that consists of depriving factors like feeling fatigued, feeling weak, and feeling discomfort at every moment of our life. It may play a huge role in our life by being part of every daily life activity that we go through daily and could even keep us weakening to the point where we feel exhausted at every moment.

There are many pains and discomforts that a person goes through in their life. They may feel sick or acquire a disease that keeps them from doing certain tasks.

Being sick or unwell is similar to a short-term sickness that affects our mind and body frequently. It may be anything that can be obtained due to eating less and completely neglecting our diets, or it could be the cause of not sleeping well or taking care of our body the way we are required to.

We may face certain obstacles in life, which may be classified from mild to extreme, and facing these obstacles and making rational decisions regarding them is something that is to be done with full control of our minds. When things get tough, our bodies should be in good shape to support our minds and be a positive component that not only helps us take the appropriate action but also helps us keep it in place.

Our bodies are safe places that simply require us to provide them with proper nutrition and care. It may be something that weakens over time, but giving it the right care from the start is something that should be implemented in our lives from an early age. This feeling of being unwell is also known as malaise, it is a feeling of discomfort or simply a feeling where a person does not feel well, even after getting an adequate amount of rest.

This feeling may come suddenly and might stay for a while before leaving, while in some other cases it may gradually increase over time and stay for a longer period, influencing the life of the affected in negative ways.

Many symptoms are connected to malaise. These may affect us daily or may suddenly affect our lives in unexpected ways. Pain, discomfort, constant illness, fatigue, and even depression could be the symptoms of this instant and continuing sickness. We may not know it, but we may stop taking proper care of ourselves at some time in our lives. We may suddenly start consuming less food or sleep when no one is around to keep an eye on us. These unrecognized habits may cause complications for both body and mind and may even lead us to the brink of forming a permanent illness of sorts or something that is temporary but its effects are everlasting.

Although the symptoms are vast and keep a person uncomfortable, the causes of such illnesses are many and can be due to various daily life activities and the common, regular routines we may have in our life. Overexertion is one of the main reasons we acquire this feeling of constant sickness.

When we try to overachieve things, we don't realize the problems this could cause later and hence we push the consequences of our actions to the back of our minds. Decreased physical activity, the time we spend doing nothing with the use of our body can get our body used to not moving and not doing anything, which may later cause fatigue and laziness, causing the body to feel weak and feverish, which isn't often the case.

Another reason for this may be jet lag, which a person may suffer through after long hours of flight. Viral infections may also be one reason why a person gets a fever, and its side effects last for a longer period. Aging may also be one reason for going through such effects. Either way, feeling unwell is like feeling unproductive to do anything.

We are not motivated enough to achieve a certain task which further demotivates us, and can harm our minds. Being able to complete a task, no matter how important or trivial it may be, is the first step toward success for many individuals, and this can encourage them to do more and gradually learn to execute these things and achieve success despite overcoming compulsions of fatigue's influence on our bodies.

Whatever the reasons may be for feeling such symptoms and feelings, it's always best for a person to maintain a balanced diet and take care of their body regularly. Wherever a person may be, they should always keep their bodies active, doing a certain task around the house, walking while on a call, or just walking, in general, is a great activity that is calming and doesn't require a lot of effort to do.

When we feel unwell, we lose a glow that we may always have on our faces or the effects that we had of it previously. That glow can be revived by taking care of our body and mind properly, not letting anything negative affect us, and taking over the thoughts in our minds.

What Is Wellness?

Wellness, as we perceive it, is known to be in good physical wealth as well as a good mental one. It can also be determined as a choice and a process in which people make decisions for their advantage, become aware of crucial and healthy options, and live a more appealing and successful lifestyle as a consequence of their physical well-being.

Wellness is constituted by what makes a person physically and mentally strong enough to do certain things and keeps them influenced sufficiently to achieve these tasks continuously. Numerous factors contribute to our well-being, as well as many habits that develop through time and aid in the development of a healthy result and lifestyle for ourselves and others around us.

- Influence is one factor that may keep a person wondering more about wellness.
- It constitutes the number one reason people start to believe in maintaining their health, which regards us keeping our body in check and also staying aware of the thoughts that go through our mind, whether their capacity is very high or low enough to prove no harm to us.
- This may help us differentiate between our thoughts and keep them in control.

Various things occur in our lives that influence wellness in our lives. They may be numerous and only work for some, but there are many more that would have a beneficial impact on someone's life and assist them in achieving their goals.

Such tasks, or challenges as we might name them, can be tackled one at a time and gently and concisely integrated into our life. When we choose to make healthy choices in our lives, we choose to live a lifestyle that includes less stress, great relationships, and happiness.

Wellness by many is only considered to be related to or linked to health. While this is not the case, many still hold a firm belief in it and acknowledge wellness to be only from a healthy viewpoint, and that belief is examined only for the healthiness of the body.

Wellness, as defined by the World Health Organization, is described as a condition of mental, physical, and social well-being rather than simply the absence of a disease or a common fever.

The environment in which we live, particularly the lifestyle that we finally establish for ourselves, impacts our well-being and speculates on whether the ways we have already implemented in our lives are the best options for us.

The different dimensions of wellness are many and since the determination of wellness is just related to the physical health of our body, it has been redefined and taken into understanding with different scenarios and also with satisfaction and the quality of life.

- Its dimensions, although many, are all related to our well-being, not only in the mind and body but also by the kind of environment or the habitat we have all around us.

- Many things have to be concisely implemented in our lives to have the sort of life that can be lived healthily and without any impending concerns.
- Many techniques that assist in having a healthy mentality together with a comfortable body are half of the happiness a person may obtain in their life, especially since they are the most crucial aspects that can impact how someone behaves, feels, and acts.
- Society, environment, screen time, and many other factors may or may not influence our lives differently. These may range from being familiar to being occasional.
- Some techniques such as mindfulness, exercise, sleeping, and diet may improve our lives and have a favorable impact on both our bodies and minds.
- Many emotions, as well as many other benefits, are inherited when we are well, or when we are successful in feeling the full force of wellness.
- When we are well, many things come into form in our life that would never be there if we were physically or psychologically ill. These things contribute to us feeling positive emotions that are capable of always keeping us happy.
- They may range from happiness to being entirely positive about everything around us, especially the things that other people may find bleak.
- When our body is physically and mentally healthy, and even when it is viewed from the perspective of the many dimensions of wellbeing, the aspects that keep us happy and positive in life will be adopted effortlessly.

These factors can have a very positive approach on our minds and bodies, and these are to be wholly appreciated since they are only acquired by keeping good care of our bodies and our mental state, and also by ensuring that we follow specific methods to keep them glowing and benefitting.

- The enjoyment of these activities in our lives, as well as our thoughts that appear to be flowing at a good level, are always what a person wants in whatever they do once they have them.
- Even when they are stressed, they wish to have a stress-free, satisfying life in which they see themselves as happy. One such way is based on our nutritious diet, which many people would want to avoid because they are unaware of the benefits or because the flavor may not be to their liking.

Wellness shots are one factor that if implemented in our life regularly may help a person brighten their day by feeling good physically which will even affect mental health more positively since both of them almost always go hand in hand.

The advantages and the reasons for taking wellness shots are many and they are always held by the people who have always practiced them:

- These benefits are only healthily acquired by such factors and prove to be very useful in many cases like weight loss, preventing weakness, or even just for glowing skin.
- The creation of wellness shots is fairly easy and also isn't time-consuming.
- Although they are known to be health boosters, something that can be taken in addition to consuming food regularly and in a healthy manner, they are known to affect a person's bodily functions, also providing important nutrients immediately as a person drinks them.
- When people have busy timetables they may not want to have such drinks since they might think of them as fairly hard to make among their working schedules, and including them at a particular time will be hard to adjust.

However, always keeping them ready in a container can help greatly.

- Having them always or even occasionally stored at the right temperature and having the recommended daily amount can help a great deal.
- If people follow this technique and keep it ready in advance, it may benefit them on a new level and also teach them to implement various other things in their life, although the first step is to be taken by them.

How Do You Know If You Are Well?

Many factors contribute to us being well and unwell and these may be classified as whatever people may think of them to be, but they come with a lot of hardships and a lot of things that we never thought could go well.

There are a lot of events and a load more situations that we face in our daily lives, they may come as unexpected or they may come to be something that we have always known and felt a certain way about.

- When a person knows they are well, they feel enlightened about all the various things that they have faced in their lives and whatever they may face in the future.

The belief of knowing that one may be okay after whatever they have been through in life is something that many look forward to and relish when they have that moment of understanding.

- Knowing that we are physically, mentally, and spiritually well is a feeling of great relief, not one that we can feel regularly but rather one that we feel when we are at a point in our life where everything is great and we have achieved something.

- It's the point where we have an understanding, an appreciation, and a known thought of having this moment and deserving it.

Another aspect of feeling well is gratefulness.

- When we are grateful for something we are grateful for everything in our life, and, hence, this keeps us doing good and makes our life easier knowing that we are grateful for everything we have and are content with it.

A comfy bed to sleep in is one expression that could relate to this aspect. Many people still think of what they would eat, how they will earn money, and whether should they sleep or not.

These questions are posed in a society where materials are scarce and earning food is like earning for the day, and then the next day is the same routine just as the previous one.

- This notion keeps a person thinking and influences them to appreciate even the smallest of things in their life, which is one factor that affects our thoughts more positively and keeps them from going astray looking at everything that is around them.

When you strive to be better and are feeling a bit down because you haven't achieved something, it means that you are trying and wanting to do better, one of the mere factors of feeling well but also something that may influence a person negatively or positively.

- We need to give our thoughts on the benefit and think about how we can do better the next time and what we can do to achieve the certain achievement that we are looking forward to.

- Thoughts like anxiety and stress should be kept away since they could demotivate a person and make them focus on things that are unnecessary rather than the necessary ones.

A person's happiness is also one element that could describe their mental well-being and could efficiently describe their mood.

- A person's happiness is a reflection of their soul, their real happiness can be defined as one where they don't need to fake it for anyone or for themselves, and at that moment they are feeling those heightened emotions of happiness and everything else combined. They are happy.
- One huge factor in determining if we are well, or if it is just a temporary moment in our lives, can be happy.
- It displays our mental as well as physical well-being and can also be a source for the start of many other things that may make a person feel elated without any concerns.

Our mental health concerns are many and should be looked at every once in a while to peek into our minds and see if the thoughts that go through them are concerning to us or could lead to problems later.

Staying aware of both what is on our minds and our surroundings and environments is an important contribution that we can give to our life. Especially when we know the dangers that prevail around us or even those that are present within us.

- It is always necessary to stay alert whenever it comes to matters of our health as well as our environment because, in the end, we are the ones making all the decisions. Whatever is good or bad in our life is going to directly affect us after all.

- Having observed this, we can know for sure that whenever we do have to take action, we base it on our mental and physical health as well as the environment that we have around us.
- These factors determine the choices we make and keep in our lives and are regularly affected by them.
- To be well is to know that you are all right mentally and physically, but also knowing that everything that surrounds you won't affect you negatively, and no matter what, you may keep smiling, and keep thinking positive thoughts all the while unknowingly living a healthy life.
- It is an agreement that (with ourselves) at this moment, even if only for a certain amount of time, we will be well.
- We will keep calm and live as happily and as positively as we can, especially when the case arises that we may be given these joys in life temporarily.
- We live a life where everything comes and goes, where everything around us is temporary and may change the next moment.
- Knowing that we are well also involves getting the right amount of sleep and food and the right amount of bodily movements.
- It involves us making friends with people we trust and are happy with and avoiding the ones that make us feel uncomfortable or insecure.
- It is being grateful in life and making the right decisions, especially with the right mind.
- Everything around us that constitutes "being well" suggests that we need to apply certain habits in our life to achieve wellness.
- A walk anywhere would be helpful.

- Exercising and meditating could be other methods and some others do not involve moving at all.
- Wellness shots, which may be taken as booster shots and kept in handy whenever one may need them.

These are the most common factors that affect our wellness, and certain others contribute equally to us being well.

Chapter 5: The Benefits of Wellness Shots

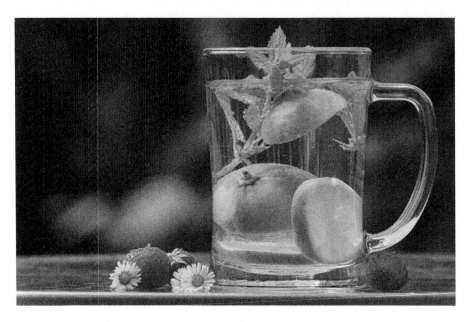

Some common wellness shots are usually heard of and implemented in different people's lives. These benefit the person equally and choosing the best out of all these is something that depends on various aspects.

Whether the person will be willing to consume them or whether they would prefer other things completely tends to depend on their will and choice. People may consume different wellness shots based on their preferences in taste, benefits, and even ingredients used, since many times the ingredients that are used in wellness shots may not be to everyone's liking.

Wellness shots have a keen kind of difference, which many other medicines or many other solutions may not have. They are more likely to benefit a person in a healthy manner and their consumption always ensures that a person stays healthy and gains the right amount of nutrients and benefits through these drinks.

When we compare them with pills, for example, we may note the difference. The pill provides relief only from pain and, in some other cases, may lead to unneeded addictions to them. While in the case of wellness shots, they may provide relief as well as various other nutrients that a person did not seek but ended up getting.

Some advantages that are common and may be found in wellness shots are:

- They increase immunity levels which benefits the overall health of the body.
- They aid in many unexpected ailments and provide relief as needed.
- They help promote weight loss in a healthy manner.
- They help in fighting chronic diseases and prevent inflation.
- They improve brain function and help a person focus.
- They provide our bodies with immeasurable amounts of nutrients and vitamins.
- They act as instant boosters for our energy levels and can help us go through a busy day more efficiently.

Overall, we can see that these wellness shots are of great advantage and have various benefits to them. These cannot be measured in front of other activities and other kinds of medicines that we may consume. Having them implemented in our lives is like implementing the various nutrients and other advantages that come with them. Having said this, wellness shots come in many kinds of different ingredients combined, and the mixtures are known to be efficient in providing healthy relief.

Therefore, having these shots and keeping them prepared in advance is one big favor we can do for ourselves, especially when we know we need the extra advantages and benefits. Listed below are the different wellness shots, which have their own unique nutrients and have their own advantages that they help in providing to the body.

Tips for Consuming Wellness Shots

- When implementing these wellness shots in our life, we must be aware of how we should be consuming them, what time we consume them, and why we consume them. Other than the fact that these wellness shots are of great help, many right methods are taken in consuming them.
- When getting ready to prepare a wellness shot, it is recommended to always keep a blender or juicer ready. These are the main pieces of equipment that are used in making the majority of wellness shots and are efficient in providing the best results.
- Wellness shots are mostly refrigerated before consumption. A time of 15 minutes or even up to one week can be given to refrigerate these drinks to prepare in advance and consume when chilled.
- The ingredients used should be fresh and natural since the number of nutrients one gets from them is a sufficient amount that helps in benefitting a person and also helps with preventing various ailments that a person suffers through.
- When starting to consume one of these shots, it is better to check any sort of allergies a person may have to an ingredient.
- It is also better to view the various benefits and start taking them for a necessary reason, whether it be for

weight loss, improving skin health, or even preventing cold and flu.

- When starting to consume these wellness shots, it is a crucial step to take them regularly and keep consuming them since this way of acquiring them provides a person with efficient results.

Conclusion

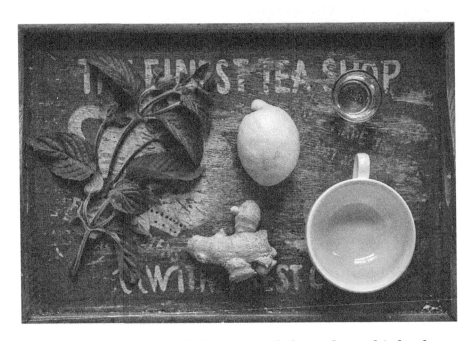

As we have read and probably learned throughout this book, we have noticed the various side effects that occur when we feel unwell constantly. We are in constant pain and sickness and may feel fatigued more than usual.

This could cause us problems both mentally and physically. Feeling this kind of daily fatigue and irritation in our body can be unbearable after some time. Even after just a few days it can become something that won't let us do specific tasks, keeps us from working, and even have us feeling weak and unmotivated.

This kind of feeling is also known as malaise, the feeling where life is just a lag of activities. Even if a person wishes to do something, they may be too unmotivated to do it and end up only thinking of doing a particular task and dwelling on the matter of how they can start and never end up actually doing it.

It's a fact that many things in today's world are easily accessible. Social media, online stores, and even online jobs keep us going, but while we are achieving the said convenience of not leaving our house and having it easy, we sort of become lazier.

There is a hint of unwillingness for us to leave the house, everything may be done online in advance or some things may not be done at all, left for later, which never seems to come. This is one of the reasons why people end up being unwell. They lose all the natural sources that keep them healthy and give them the natural vitamins that only such natural resources can.

Being well, on the other hand, is a huge accomplishment since we are allowing our body to feel happier and helping it build more confidence with gratitude, calmness, and perhaps time in our lives where we may have a lot to achieve, but we are content. This could be one way of identifying a person's wellness.

Knowing that whatever we have achieved in life is satisfactory for us and knowing that whatever we achieve could be something we look forward to with a positive mindset and work hard towards, we will end up achieving anyway. It's crucial for us to always be present at the moment every single moment of our lives. It's also crucial to keep analyzing ourselves and our behavior. We may not know it, but our observation of ourselves can speak volumes about how we are and what we feel.

A lifestyle that speaks volumes about us is also important since it determines how we take care of ourselves and the others around us, including how we like to keep things and our preferences. The instant mood change makes us prefer doing nothing rather than doing something and creates more problems that a person going through something may prefer to not address and hence completely give up on the task at hand.

This person may not be well. Many emotions and other dimensions are associated with wellness. Many of these enter our lives in numerous forms and others may be more evident and instantly show a person's status of well-being.

Now, as we talk about wellness and its different aspects, we can also seek to find methods or techniques that help bring wellness into our lives and keep us doing good and staying refreshed at times when we may not feel like it. Walking, sports of any kind, or even some nature-related activities help relax both our minds and body.

They keep us physically fit and mentally stimulated. While many people may love to implement such activities in their life, their busy schedules may not allow enough time to implement them or practice them. They may instead do something else that easily fits into their busy schedules.

Wellness shots could be made a part of our daily routines, not necessarily all the shots out there, but some that may benefit us according to our body's specific nutrient and vitamin needs. We may not find them suitable to our taste, or they may be sufficiently hard to make.

While this may be the case, wellness shots have the easiest recipes and are very convenient to make. The maximum time a wellness shot may take to make is 15 minutes. The ingredients that are added are natural, and their nourishing nutrients are the same when added to the mixture and when taken out to consume.

Wellness shots are boosters that give out energy and replenishment, aiding us by helping our skin glow, keeping our body strong, aiding in other pains like aging and stomachaches, and providing relief after consumption. These may also benefit us by providing us with a sufficient amount of sleep due to the active ingredients present in the recipes.

This is something crucial to observe and seek since taking care of our health is a necessary factor in our lives and knowing what can cause us relief and pain is the knowledge we should aim to have. It's not always the case that people may find instant relief with these shots. They may believe it to be a bluff and miss the importance of keeping them in their lives.

It isn't always true that everything may provide us with harm if we consume it without the right guidance. Sometimes the right guidance can also be the recipes that can help us nourish our diet and add to it by providing our body with an extra amount of supplement.

Taking care of our bodies and keeping our life in check is our responsibility, no one else may care. It is our responsibility to look after ourselves the way we would look after someone else. We may be all for our loved ones to be safe and comfortable and implement healthiness in their lives.

Well, this behavior, although we do it for the benefit of others, should also be done for the benefit of ourselves. We should take care of ourselves and keep guarding ourselves against anything that threatens our immunity or thoughts negatively. Our wellness is our priority and its safekeeping falls into our hands, anything that may provide harm should be removed from our lives.

It could be anything from our surrounding environment or something that could be threatening us mentally. Methods such as wellness shots should be taken and implemented, so that we may have extra nutrients and extra energy in our daily life.

- and diet may improve our lives and have a favorable impact on both our bodies and minds.
- Many emotions, as well as many other benefits, are inherited when we are well, or when we are successful in feeling the full force of wellness.
- When we are well, many things come into form in our life that would never be there if we were physically or psychologically ill. These things contribute to us feeling positive emotions that are capable of always keeping us happy.
- They may range from happiness to being entirely positive about everything around us, especially the things that other people may find bleak.
- When our body is physically and mentally healthy, and even when it is viewed from the perspective of the many dimensions of wellbeing, the aspects that keep us happy and positive in life will be adopted effortlessly.

These factors can have a very positive approach to our minds and bodies, and these are to be wholly appreciated since they are only acquired by keeping good care of our bodies and our mental state, also by ensuring that we follow specific methods to keep them glowing and benefitting.

- The enjoyment of these activities in our lives, as well as our thoughts that appear to be flowing at a good level, are always what a person wants in whatever they do once they have them.
- Even when they are stressed, they wish to have a stress-free, satisfying life in which they see themselves as happy. One such way is based on our nutritious diet, which many people would want to avoid because they are unaware of the benefits or because the flavor may not be to their liking.

Wellness shots are one factor which if implemented in our life regularly may help a person brighten their day by feeling good physically which will even affect the mental health more positively since the both of them almost always go hand in hand. The advantages and the reasons for taking wellness shots are many and they are always held by the people who have always practiced them.

- These benefits are only healthily acquired by such factors and prove to be very useful in many cases like weight loss, preventing weakness, or even just for glowing skin.
- The creation of wellness shots is fairly easy and also isn't time consuming.
- Although they are known to be health boosters, something that can be taken in addition to consuming food regularly and in a healthy manner, they are known to affect a person's bodily functions, also providing important nutrients immediately as a person drinks them.
- When people have busy timetables they may not want to have such drinks since they might think of them as fairly hard to make among their working schedules, and including them at a particular time will be hard to adjust. However, always keeping them ready in a container can help greatly.
- Having them always or even occasionally stored at the right temperature and having the recommended daily amount can help a great deal.
- If people follow this technique and keep it ready in advance, it may benefit them on a new level and also teach them to implement various other things in their life, although the first step is to be taken by them.

How does one know if they are well?

Many factors contribute to us being well and unwell and these may be classified as whatever people may think of them to be, but they come with a lot of hardships and a lot of things that we never thought could go well. There are a lot of events and a load more situations that we face in our daily lives, they may come as unexpected or they may come to be something that we have always known and felt a certain way about.

- When a person knows they are well, they feel enlightened about all the various things that they have faced in their lives and whatever they may face in the future.

The belief of knowing that one may be okay after whatever they have been through in life is something that many look forward to and relish when they have that moment of understanding.

- Knowing that we are physically, mentally, and spiritually well is a feeling of great relief, not one that we can feel regularly but rather one that we feel when we are at a point in our life where everything is great and we have achieved something.
- It's the point where we have an understanding, an appreciation, and a known thought of having this moment and deserving it.

Another aspect of feeling well is gratefulness.

- When we are grateful for something we are grateful for everything in our life, and, hence, this keeps us doing good and makes our life easier knowing that we are grateful for everything we have and are content with it.

A comfy bed to sleep in is one expression that could relate to this aspect. Many people still think of what they would eat, how they will earn money, and should they sleep or not? These questions are posed in a society where materials are scarce and earning food is like earning for the day, and then the next day is the same routine just as the previous one.

- This notion keeps a person thinking and influences them to appreciate even the smallest of things in their life, which is one factor that affects our thoughts more positively and keeps them from going astray looking at everything that is around them.

When you strive to be better and are feeling a bit down because you haven't achieved something, it means that you are trying and wanting to do better, one of the mere factors of feeling well but also something that may influence a person negatively or positively.

- We need to give our thoughts on the benefit and think about how we can do better the next time and what we can do to achieve the certain achievement that we are looking forward to.
- Thoughts like anxiety and stress should be kept away since they could demotivate a person and make them focus on things that are unnecessary rather than the ones that are necessary.

A person's happiness is also one element that could describe their mental well-being and could efficiently describe their mood.

- A person's happiness is a reflection of their soul, their real happiness can be defined as one where they don't need to fake it for anyone or for themselves, and at that moment they are feeling those heightened emotions of happiness and everything else combined. They are happy.

- One huge factor in determining if we are well, or if it is just a temporary moment in our lives, can be happiness.
- It displays our mental as well as physical well-being and can also be a source for the start of many other things that may make a person feel elated without any concerns.

Our mental health concerns are many and should be looked at every once in a while to peek into our mind and see if the thoughts that go through it are concerning to us or could lead to problems later.

Staying aware of both what is on our minds and our surroundings and environments is an important contribution that we can give to our life. Especially when we know the dangers that prevail around us, or even those that are present within us.

- It is always necessary to stay alert whenever it comes to matters of our health as well as our environment because, in the end, we are the ones making all the decisions. Whatever is good or bad in our life is going to directly affect us after all.
- Having observed this, we can know for sure that whenever we do have to take action, we base it off on our mental and physical health as well as the environment that we have around.
- These factors determine the choices we make and keep in our lives and are regularly affected by them.
- To be well is to know that you are alright mentally and physically, but also knowing that everything that surrounds you won't affect you negatively, and no matter what, you may keep smiling, keep thinking of positive thoughts all the while unknowingly living a healthy life.

- It is an agreement that (with ourselves) at this moment, even if only for a certain amount of time, we will be well.
- We will keep calm and live as happily and as positively as we can, especially when the case arises that we may be given these joys in life temporarily.
- We live a life where everything comes and goes, where everything around us is temporary and may change the next moment.
- Knowing that we are well also involves us getting the right amount of sleep and food and the right amount of bodily movements.
- It involves us making friends with people we trust and are happy with and avoiding the ones that make us feel uncomfortable or insecure.
- It is being grateful in life and making the right decisions, especially with the right mind.
- Everything around us that constitutes being well suggests that we need to apply certain habits in our life to achieve wellness.
- A walk anywhere would be helpful.
- Exercising and meditating could be other methods and some others which do not involve moving at all.
- Wellness shots, which may be taken as booster shots and kept in handy whenever one may need them.

These are the most common factors that affect our wellness, and there are certain others which contribute equally in us being well.

References

Pappadopulos, E. (n.d.). *What is Wellness? | Pfizer.*
https://www.pfizer.com/health-wellness/wellness/what-is-
wellness#:~:text=Wellness%20is%20the%20act%20of

Glassman, K. (2019, August 22). *What are wellness shots —
and are they actually worth it? |* TODAY.com.
https://www.today.com/health/wellness-shots-what-are-
real-health-benefits-t159321